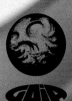

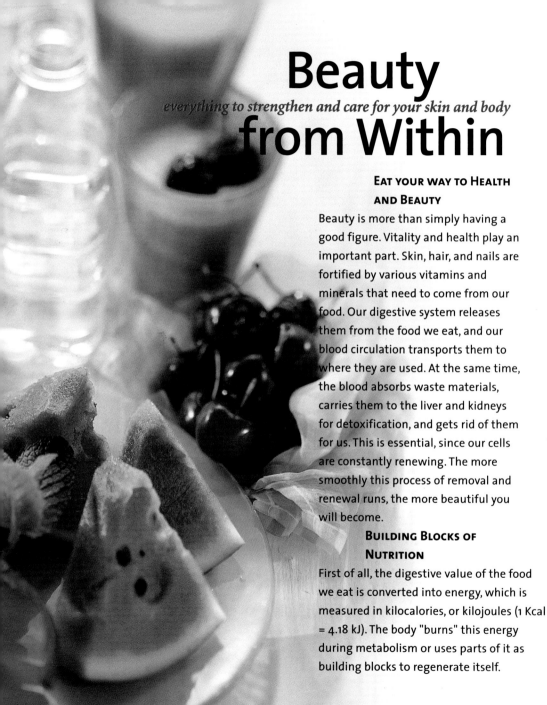

Beauty
everything to strengthen and care for your skin and body
from Within

EAT YOUR WAY TO HEALTH AND BEAUTY

Beauty is more than simply having a good figure. Vitality and health play an important part. Skin, hair, and nails are fortified by various vitamins and minerals that need to come from our food. Our digestive system releases them from the food we eat, and our blood circulation transports them to where they are used. At the same time, the blood absorbs waste materials, carries them to the liver and kidneys for detoxification, and gets rid of them for us. This is essential, since our cells are constantly renewing. The more smoothly this process of removal and renewal runs, the more beautiful you will become.

BUILDING BLOCKS OF NUTRITION

First of all, the digestive value of the food we eat is converted into energy, which is measured in kilocalories, or kilojoules (1 Kcal = 4.18 kJ). The body "burns" this energy during metabolism or uses parts of it as building blocks to regenerate itself.

These building blocks are:

* Carbohydrates are the principal component of fruit, vegetables, and grains. Carbohydrate foods also provide fibre, water-soluble vitamins, and minerals. However, some carbohydrates also contain fast-releasing sugar, which, if taken to excess, can make us tired and lethargic.
* Protein is a building block in our cells. It is present in enzymes, hormones, and antibodies, and carries our genetic materials. It is needed constantly for cell renewal. Protein is found in fish, meat, eggs, dairy products, cereals, and grains.
* Fat is a constituent of hormones and bile acids. It carries fat-soluble vitamins, and is a building component in cell walls – and thus in our skin. Unsaturated fatty acids are vital to health, and are contained in good-quality, cold-pressed oils. The hidden fats in meat products, cakes and biscuits – which taste delicious – are tricky, though, and will settle around your waist, just like a 'spare tyre'.
* Fibre can help banish sluggishness. It consists of plant cellulose, which your body cannot use, and so it contains no calories. Fibre is present mainly in fruit, vegetables, and grains. It keeps us "regular"; in other words, it makes sure that waste products are quickly expelled. And fibre fills us up without producing weight gain.

THE LITTLE THINGS THAT MEAN A LOT

The body is unable to produce a lot of the active substances that monitor and control our metabolism; we need to absorb them from the food we eat. And although we need only the tiniest quantities of these substances, we still often do not have enough of them. You can read more about this on the next page.

* Minerals are the building blocks for bones, teeth, hair, and blood – but they also regulate the central metabolic processes, and maintain our inner balance.
* Vitamins are involved in every single metabolic process, and play a decisive role in processing foods in our diet, i.e. they help us to produce energy. They strengthen our immune system, regulate our mineral balance, and control cell regulation.
* Although so-called 'bio-active' substances (phytochemicals, or plant chemicals) are not essential, they do play a key role in keeping us healthy and feeling good. They are created in the metabolic process of plants, so are present in fruit, vegetables, and cereals. Many of them not only help to prevent circulatory problems and atherosclerosis, but also protect the cells against environmental damage.

NUTRIENT	EFFECT
Vitamin D	Prevents osteoporosis by stimulating the body to absorb more calcium
Vitamin E	Antioxidant – protects against free radicals, keeps tissues elastic, stimulates the circulation
Vitamin B_1	Strengthens nerves and muscles
Vitamin B_2	For protein metabolism, cell division, nervous system, helps with PMS and morning sickness
Vitamin B_{12}	Essential for cell division and blood formation
Niacin	For smooth skin and good nerves, and to utilize energy
Pantothenic acid	Promotes skin and hair renewal, aids healing
Folic acid	For cell division and formation, formation of blood cells, immune system
Iron	Formation of blood cells, healthy skin, shiny hair, hard fingernails
Selenium	For healthy skin and nails. Detoxifies
Zinc	For strong hair and healthy skin, aids healing and the immune system, improves sensuality
Iodine	For a properly functioning metabolism, helps keep a slim figure
Calcium	For strong bones, teeth, nails, and hair; benefits the nerves
Silicic acid	Firms tissues, and strengthens skin and hair
Lactic acid	Beneficial to the flora in the gut, and the immune system, aids iron absorption
Omega-3-fatty acids	Aid circulation and help maintain a healthy heart
Gamma-linoleic acid	For healthy, firm skin
Carotenoids	Boosts the immune system. A precursor of vitamin A, beta-carotene is good for smooth, healthy skin

Found In

Oily fish, egg yolk, butter. Produced by the skin in the sun

High-quality plant oils, especially wheatgerm oil, margarine, fish, grains, and nuts

Wholewheat products, yeast, potatoes, pulses

Wholewheat products, fish, sea fish, cabbage, leeks, beans

Meat, fish, dairy products, foods containing lactic acid, yeast extract

Wholewheat products, meat, fish, pulses, potatoes

Liver, yeast, mushrooms, wholewheat products

Raw green vegetables, nuts, seeds, yeast, oranges, mango

Meat, fish, millet, green vegetables, dried fruit, nuts

Fish (especially tuna, bloater and herring), whole grains, vegetables, mushrooms

Brewer's yeast, pulses, cheese, liver, nuts, sea vegetables, oysters

Sea fish, iodized salt, good quantities in sea vegetables

Dairy products, especially hard cheese

Whole grains, especially millet, oats, barley

Products containing lactic acid: sauerkraut, pickled gherkins, yogurt, kefir, whey, buttermilk, cheese, salami, olives, soy sauce

Oily fish (herring, salmon), linseed and rapeseed oil

Plant oils (borage, sunflower, thistle, linseed), margarine, avocado, fish

Good quantities in yellow, red, and green fruits and vegetables, such as apricots, pumpkin, and broccoli

Beauty

everything for beauty

Basics

THE WONDERFUL POWERS OF NATURAL OILS

Fats are made of glycerine, and three fatty acids, some of which are essential; we need them to stay alive. They are present mainly in plant oils. If the oil is cold-pressed, the sensitive substances and the delicate aroma of the field products are retained. Remember: polyunsaturated fats should never be heated to a high heat, so use a small amount of olive oil (rich in monounsaturated fats) for cooking; then add a tablespoon of cold-pressed polyunsaturated oil just before eating. The following oils are especially beneficial:

* Linseed oil – contains good amounts of omega-3 fatty acids, is yellow in colour, and has a slightly bitter aroma. It goes well with strong flavours.

* Rapeseed oil – also contains plenty of omega-3 fatty acids, and has a fresh flavour; good in salads.

* Wheatgerm oil – has an exceptionally high proportion of vitamin E, a grainy-nutty flavour, and goes well in sweet dishes.

* Olive oil – consists mainly of monounsaturated fatty acids that prevent the arteries from clogging.

* Borage oil – contains a good amount of gamma linoleic acid which is effective against eczema and general skin irritations. Use by the teaspoonful.

* Black cumin oil – contains polyunsaturated fatty acids and minerals that are effective against allergic and inflammatory symptoms. The oil has a spicy, oriental aroma.

These oils are the only ones used in this book. They are obtainable from health-food shops, or you can order them from the address at the back of this book. Remember: store these valuable oils in the refrigerator, and use within a few days.

WATER FOR CRISPNESS

Our bodies consist of at least two-thirds water; younger people have a little more, older ones a little less. Water dissolves and transports the water-soluble nutrients in our body. It balances temperature and removes hazardous materials. Water makes the skin firm and smooth. Our bodies need between 1.5 and 2 litres (2 $\frac{1}{2}$ and 3 $\frac{1}{2}$ pints) of water a day, and more in warm weather or if we are performing hard physical work or sport. Do not be afraid of tap water: it is subject to strict regulations.

Fresh from the Sea

Salt water contains lots of minerals, some of which are rare on dry land, such as iodine, iron, calcium, magnesium, fluoride, and zinc. Sea vegetables, mussels, and crustaceans filter these minerals out of the sea, and concentrate them.

✵ Nori is a sea vegetable, available roasted, shredded into fine leaves for use in sushi. It is delicate, slightly spicy yet tasty, and may be soaked before eating, although this is not essential. Nori is high in protein, and contains large amounts of vitamins A and C, and plenty of calcium and iron.

✵ Arame is a brown sea vegetable that is cut into thin strips, and is bursting with iodine and calcium. Arame contains more iron and vitamin B12 than meat, and is therefore ideal for a meat-free diet. Arame is soaked for 5 minutes before cooking, when it will double in volume.

✵ Oily saltwater fish such as salmon, tuna, mackerel, and herring contain large amounts of highly beneficial omega-3 fatty acids. They also contain good quantities of protein and iodine.

✵ Prawns, shrimp, and mussels are delicate reserves of zinc, iron, selenium, and fluoride. RECOMMENDATION: Use organic produce wherever possible. If you wish to avoid genetically modified (GM) foods, read any labels with care and select certified organic produce, as this is not produced from GM ingredients.

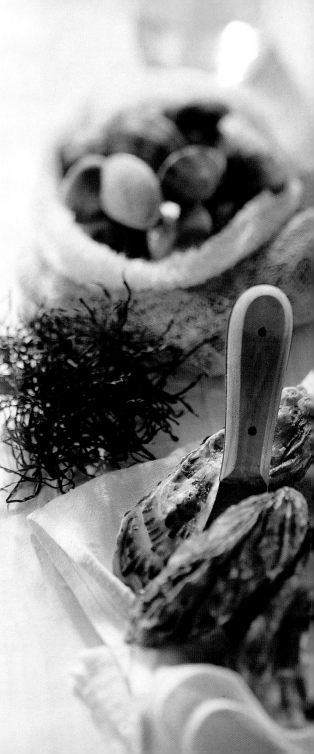

Natural
for healthy-looking skin and shiny hair
Skincare

Balsam for the Skin

Our skin breathes through its pores. It eliminates waste products and is able to absorb beneficial substances. Cold-pressed oils, fruit, vegetables, milk, and milk products contain substances that affect the skin in a number of different ways.

Packs are the most intensive way of influencing what happens to the skin. They can be made from fresh ingredients, applied to the face and around the neck while still fresh, then covered with a moist cloth and left to work for 20–30 minutes. The benefits are even greater if you can lie down and relax while the pack works. Rinse off the pack with plenty of lukewarm water, and apply a nourishing cream.

The four following packs are intended for use on four different skin types. They are all so gentle that they may safely be applied once or twice a week.

For any Skin Type: Peach Mask

A ripe, aromatic, fragrant peach is the best. Peel and chop the peach, and mash with a fork. Refreshes and smoothes.

For Dry Skin: Avocado Mask

Peel 1 ripe avocado, and purée with a few drops of lemon juice and 1 teaspoon of borage oil. Nourishes and revitalizes.

For Greasy Skin: Cucumber (or Sauerkraut) Mask

Wash and peel the cucumber, and grate into thin slices. Refreshes and smoothes the skin. You could also use freshly prepared sauerkraut (from a delicatessen), which is astringent and anti-inflammatory.

For Tired Skin: Swedish Mask

Drain 3 tablespoons of low-fat quark, and combine with 1 tablespoon of lemon juice, 1 tablespoon of whey or buttermilk, and 1 teaspoon of wheatgerm oil, stirring until smooth. Revitalizes and nourishes.

Skincare for the Body

If you would like to do something to benefit the skin on your whole body, a combination of massage and bath is ideal. The temperature of the bath water should be between 37°C and 39°C (98.6°F and 102.2°F). Do not spend more than 15–20 minutes in the bath: too long, and a bath that is too hot, will dry the skin rather than care for it. While you are in the bath, soak a face cloth in the water and place it on your face. Do this several times. This opens the pores and helps to cleanse the skin. Good tip: after your bath, spend half an hour on your bed with a face pack. Incidentally, cold-pressed oils, especially wheatgerm, sesame, and olive oil, are wonderful for the skin – and contain no additives. Borage oil is especially good for dry, irritable skin.

For Dry Skin
Before bathing, massage your whole body, from top to toe, with wheatgerm oil, working from the extremities toward the heart. Then run your bath, and add 3 litres (5 pints) of buttermilk or milk.

For Greasy, Impure Skin
Stand in the shower and massage your body with wheat bran, or pour 500 ml (20 fl oz) of

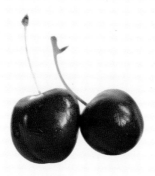

fruit vinegar into the bath water.

Strength for Your Hair
Your hair is nourished from the roots. Central heating, sun, and cold are bad for the hair, turning it dry and brittle. Apply a nourishing pack from time to time – it works like magic. Prewash your hair, then apply the lukewarm pack to your hair, avoiding your scalp but paying particular care to the roots. Then put on a shower cap, wrap a towel around your head to keep it warm, and leave the pack to work for at least 1 hour. Afterward wash your hair thoroughly with a mild shampoo.

Herb Oil for the Hair
Pour 250 ml (10 fl oz) of cold-pressed olive oil over 2–3 sprigs of thyme, 1 sprig of rosemary, and 1/2 a handful of birch leaves (as a loose-leaf tea from the pharmacy or health-food store). Place the concoction in a dark, cool place for between 1 and 4 weeks. Pass the oil through a strainer and squeeze out the herbs. Measure out the required amount before applying, then heat slightly.

Egg and Oil Pack
Depending on the length of your hair, beat 1–2 egg yolks with 1–2 teaspoons of cold-pressed wheatgerm oil. Heat the mixture until lukewarm and rub into the tips of your hair.

Power
wellbeing and relaxation at home
Week

SPOIL YOURSELF!

You don't have the time or money for a week at a spa? Then spoil yourself at home – using the recipes in this book. You should also do something for your body at the same time. Go swimming, cycling, or jogging. Spend 15 minutes a day doing some exercises. And, as a special gesture, treat yourself to a visit to the beauty salon. A massage followed by a steam bath or sauna will also do you good.

MINI SPA

Of course, you can't expect miracles in just a week, but it can be a new beginning. Incorporate some of the things you do in this week in your everyday life: drink lots of water, eat lots of fruit and vegetables, use a minimum of fat in your cooking, but make sure you do not miss out on the valuable fats. You will find that this short "cure" is a culinary delight. You will not be hungry: you can eat as many raw vegetables and berries, apples and citrus fruit as you like for the duration of the cure. But take care not to spend the whole day "grazing" – have three good meals a day, and maybe a snack in the morning or afternoon. Invite a friend to share a fondue with you on the Saturday, and serve Crunchy Melon Quark (page 19) for dessert.

DRINK YOURSELF BEAUTIFUL

Drink as much herbal and green tea as you like. You may have about two cups of ordinary tea and coffee per day, adding a little low-fat milk and cane sugar or honey – if you need it! If you don't like pure mineral water, add a "spritzer" of apple or lemon juice. And what about alcohol? Well, it's bad news for your looks, but it can definitely add to an atmosphere: you may have a glass of dry champagne at the beginning of your cure. But spare yourself on the Sunday: make sure you get lots of sleep, go for a swim and a sauna, have a soak, and put a pack on your skin and hair to motivate yourself for the week. That's not to say you must follow our suggestions to the letter: you could have a bowl of muesli and a drink in the morning, then one cold and one hot main meal of your choice later in the day. Or cook double the amount, and eat half on two days.

Menu Planner for the Week

Monday

* Happy Hour
* Cabbage and Apple Salad
* Beef Chilli with Avocado, Millet Porridge

Tuesday

* 1 slice of wholewheat bread, Whey and Mocha Mix to drink
* Bean and Shrimp Salad, with 1 slice of wholewheat bread
* Turkey Breast with Chicory

Wednesday

* Balsam Muesli with Cider Vinegar Cooler
* Choco Risotto
* Boiled New Potatoes with Power Quark

Thursday

* Melon Fruit Purée with Barley Water
* Dry-cured Beef Sandwich
* Green Ratatouille

Friday

* Orange and Carrot Quark
* Black Pesto Sandwich
* Carrot and Millet Spaghetti

Saturday

* Mild Six-grain Muesli
* Crunchy Melon Quark
* Chinese Fondue, with Grapefruit and Raw Carrot Salad

Sunday

* Fruit Salad with Grapes and a Soft Green Drink
* Catfish Cevice, followed by fruit of your choice
* Artichokes with Avocado Dip; Lamb Noisettes with Vegetables

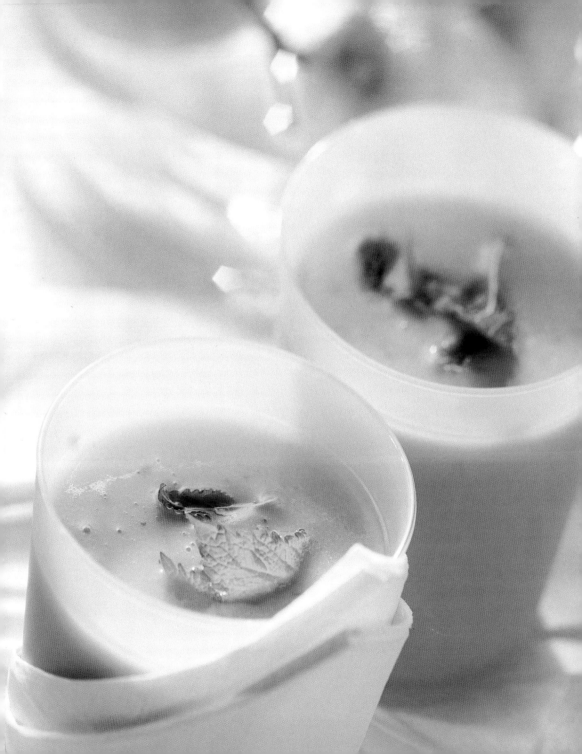

Soft

light and creamy for

Green

a little extra energy

Drink

Serves two: · 1 small, soft avocado · 2 sprigs of lemon balm · 4 tbsp lemon juice · 250 ml (10 fl oz) pear juice · 1 tsp borage oil (also known as star flower oil) · water

Halve the avocado, remove the stone, and scrape out the flesh with a spoon. Wash and shake dry the lemon balm, and remove the leaves from the stalks. Purée the avocado, lemon balm, lemon and pear juice, and the borage oil using a hand-held mixer, and dilute to taste with ice-cold water.

power

PER PORTION: 205 kcal • 2 g protein • 13 g fat • 24 g carbohydrate

Barley
lifts the mood and counters water retention
Water

For two drinks: · 60 g (2 oz) pearl barley · 1.5 litres (2¹/₂ pints) water · juice of 1 orange or other type of fruit

Wash the barley, and bring to a boil in the water. Cover with a lid and simmer for 30 minutes. Pass through a strainer. Leave the liquid to cool, then place in the refrigerator. Combine with the fruit juice, and drink well chilled.

PER DRINK: 120 kcal • 4 g protein • 1 g fat • 24 g carbohydrate

Whey and
detoxifying and aids digestion
Mocca Mix

Serves two: · 500 ml (20 fl oz) whey · 1 tbsp espresso granules · 1 tsp cocoa powder · 1 tbsp brewer's yeast · 3 tbsp cane sugar

Combine the whey, espresso and cocoa powders, yeast, and cane sugar in a blender. Shake until everything has dissolved. Add 1 small banana for a milder flavour.

PER DRINK: 85 kcal • 3 g protein • 0 g fat • 19 g carbohydrate

Cider Vinegar

cleanses from within

Cooler

Serves two: · 250 ml (10 fl oz) apple juice · 250 ml (10 fl oz) spa water · 4 tbsp cider vinegar · 1 tbsp honey

Combine the apple juice, water, vinegar, and honey; then mix well until the ingredients have dissolved. Best sipped at room temperature.

PER DRINK: 100 kcal • 0 g protein • 0 g fat • 26 g carbohydrate

Sea Buckthorn

with lots of vitamin C and beta-carotene

Cobbler

Serves two: · 80 ml (3 fl oz) buckthorn juice with honey · 300 ml (12 fl oz) freshly squeezed orange juice · 1 tsp borage or buckthorn seed oil · 1 tbsp wheatgerm

Place the buckthorn juice, orange juice, oil, and wheatgerm in a mixer. Beat well at the highest speed, then pour the cobbler into tall glasses and serve immediately.

PER DRINK: 105 kcal • 2 g protein • 3 g fat • 15 g carbohydrate

Aromatic

stimulating and skin-friendly

Muesli

Peel the grapefruit or oranges with a sharp knife, removing the white pith as well. Slice the grapefruit or oranges into quarters, and remove the white skin from the middle. Cut the quarters into slices, saving the juice in a bowl.

Serves two:
1 pink grapefruit or
2 oranges
1 ripe baby pineapple
40 g (1¹/₂ oz) flaked millet
2 tbsp wheatgerm
100 ml (4 fl oz) multi-vitamin juice

Peel the pineapple, cut lengthwise into quarters, and remove the core. Cut into bite-size pieces, saving the juice in a bowl. Place the chopped fruit and juice, flaked millet, wheatgerm, and multi-vitamin juice in a bowl, and mix. Divide the muesli between two dishes and serve.

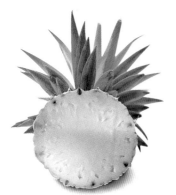

Pineapple

Pineapple contains large amounts of bromeline, which breaks down protein. It is diuretic, sudorific, and cleanses the skin. However, this applies only for fresh pineapple. You can, of course, use quarter of a standard fruit instead of a baby one.

PER PORTION:

205 kcal

5 g protein

2 g fat

42 g carbohydrate

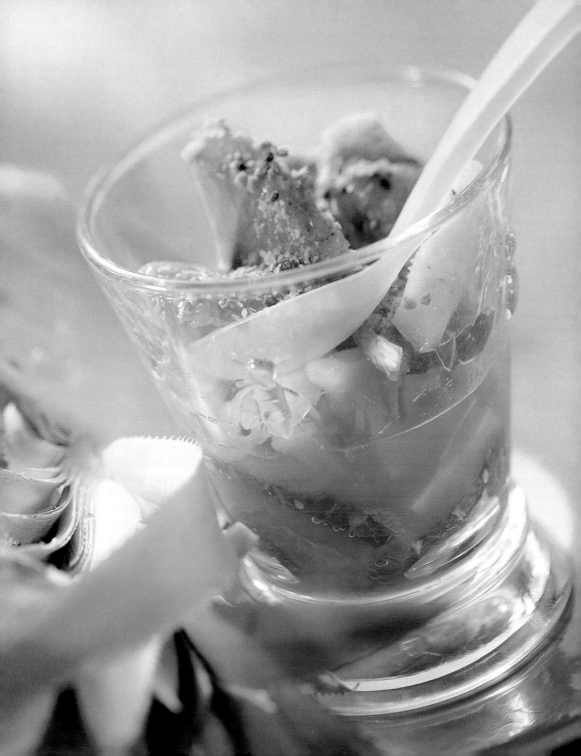

Mild

with bio-active pollen granulate

Six-grain Muesli

Serves two: · **8 each dried apricots and dried plums · 60 g (2 oz) six-grain cereal mix · 500 ml (20 fl oz) whey · 2 tbsp honey · 2 tbsp sesame seeds**

Wash the apricots and plums, and cut into small pieces. Bring the grain and fruit to a boil in 300 ml (12 fl oz) of whey. Set aside, then add the honey followed by the remaining whey. Allow the muesli to cool. Stir in the sesame seeds and serve.

PER PORTION: 405 kcal • 8 g protein • 4 g fat • 87 g carbohydrate

Happy Hour

with lots of oats and yogurt

Serves two: · **50 g (1³/₄ oz) buckwheat · 2 apples · 2 tbsp oat bran · 5 tbsp oats flakes · 500 g (18 oz) probiotic yogurt · 1 tsp borage oil · 3–4 tbsp maple syrup**

Dry-fry the buckwheat in a nonstick pan over medium heat. Wash and dry the apples, then grate them coarsely (do not peel). Combine with the oat bran, oat flakes, yogurt, borage oil, and maple syrup. Divide between two bowls, and serve.

PER PORTION: 490 kcal • 14 g protein • 13 g fat • 81 g carbohydrate

Crunchy
with protein-rich Special K
Melon Quark

Place the quark in a bowl. Add the buckthorn and orange juice, and beat well for a few minutes with a hand-held mixer. Add the yeast flakes and wheatgerm, and stir until smooth.

Wash and peel the carrot, then grate coarsely. Stir the grated carrot into the quark. Chop the melon and add to the quark. Add the Special K (or any other low-sugar, crunchy cereal, such as Corn Flakes). Spoon the quark into serving bowls and serve immediately.

Serves two:

250 g (9 oz) low-fat quark
6 tbsp sweet buckthorn juice
50 ml (1³/₄ fl oz) orange juice
1 tbsp yeast flakes
1 tbsp wheatgerm
1 young carrot
300 g (10 oz) melon (peeled)
6–8 tbsp Special K

Power pack for the skin

Wheatgerm contains vitamins E, B1, B6, and folic acid, as well as magnesium, iron, and zinc. Raw grains contain phytin, which hinders mineral absorption, so the grain should be soaked and boiled first. Flower pollen contains concentrated nutrients, enzymes, and bio-active substances. Probiotic yogurt contains active lactic acid bacteria which regenerate "good" bacteria – but only if you eat the yogurt regularly.

PER PORTION:

270 kcal

25 g protein

4 g fat

35 g carbohydrate

power

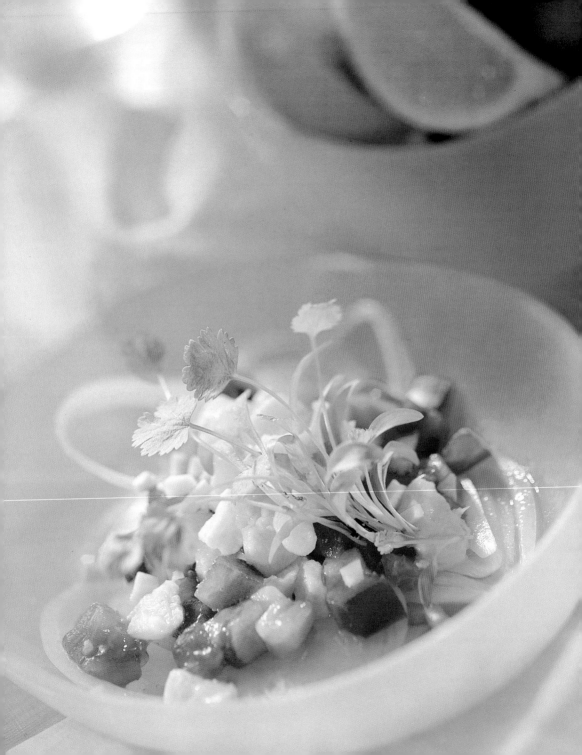

Catfish

with marinated, raw fish

Cevice

First make the marinade. Mix the lime juice and vinegar. Wash the fish and pat dry with paper towels. Cut into small pieces. Place the fish in the marinade, turning occasionally.

Wash and halve the tomatoes, remove the stalks and cores, and dice. Pour the seeds and juice over the fish. Peel the onions and slice thinly. Wash the herbs and shake dry. Remove the leaves from the stalks, and chop them finely. Peel and finely chop the ginger.

Spread the onion slices over a plate, followed by the diced tomato and the fish, and sprinkle with the herbs. Sprinkle each layer with salt, pepper, the marinade, and the oil, and top with the chopped ginger. Serve with bread.

Serves two:

juice of 1 lime
2 tbsp cider vinegar
200 g (7 oz) catfish fillets
2 beef tomatoes
2 onions
bunch of coriander or Italian parsley
piece of ginger, about the size of a walnut
1 tsp black cumin oil
sea salt and black pepper

Bounty from the Sea

The more natural the state of the fish and vegetables you eat, the better it is for you. Seeds provide fibre, and cleanse from within. The tomato's best nutrients are right below the skin, and fish "cooked" in citrus juice contains iodine and omega-3 fatty acid in their natural state.

PER PORTION:

150 kcal

19 g protein

5 g fat

8 g carbohydrate

Asparagus and
with spicy nori
Mushroom Carpaccio

Serves two:

6 tbsp cider vinegar

1 tbsp horseradish, freshly grated or paste

2 tbsp thistle oil

2 tbsp soy sauce

black pepper

6 tbsp water or white wine

250 g (9 oz) thick, white asparagus

100 g (4 oz) large mushrooms

2 large nori leaves

1 tbsp sesame seeds

To make the marinade, stir together the vinegar, horseradish, oil, soy sauce, pepper, and water or white wine. Wash and trim the asparagus. Peel carefully, then slice thinly. Trim the mushrooms, wash quickly, and cut into thin slices.

Cut the nori leaves into 4 cm (1½ in) slices. Line two large plates with half the sliced nori leaves, and sprinkle over a little of the marinade. Then divide the sliced asparagus, mushrooms, and the remaining sliced nori leaves between the plates, and sprinkle over the remaining marinade.

Dry-fry the sesame seeds in a nonstick pan, and sprinkle over the carpaccio. Leave to stand for 30 minutes, then serve with fresh rye sourdough bread.

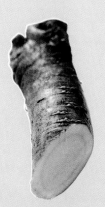

Horseradish

Contains mustard oil, which has natural antibiotic properties that support the stomach acid. It also stimulates the digestive juices. It contains even more vitamin C than capsicum.

PER PORTION:

160 kcal

5 g protein

10 g fat

8 g carbohydrate

power

Roast Beef

with rocket and pumpkin seeds

Carpaccio

To make the marinade, place the pumpkin seed and wheatgerm oils, orange juice, salt, pepper, and mustard powder in a bowl, and beat well.

Thoroughly wash the rocket, pick over, and drain well in a strainer.

Divide half the rocket between 2 plates, and sprinkle over a little of the marinade. Then arrange the roast beef and remaining rocket leaves on top, and sprinkle over the remaining marinade.

Coarsely chop the pumpkin seeds and sprinkle over the roast beef. Leave to stand for about 30 minutes, then serve with ciabatta or baguette.

Serves two:

2 tbsp pumpkin seed oil
1 tbsp wheatgerm oil
100 ml (4 fl oz) orange juice
sea salt
black pepper
1 tsp mustard powder (or hot mustard)
100 g (4 oz) rocket
150 g (5 oz) roast beef, thinly sliced
2 tbsp pumpkin seeds

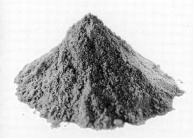

Mustard Powder

This is made of ground mustard seeds, and adds a gentle spiciness to salad dressings without adding acidity. Mustard aids digestion, is antibacterial, and promotes blood supply to tissues. It is good for indigestion. You can use ready-made mustard as a substitute.

PER PORTION:

340 kcal

23 g protein

23 g fat

11 g carbohydrate

power

Artichoke with
with basil and black cumin oil
Avocado Dip

Wash the artichokes. Break off the stalks, remove the outer leaves, and cut off any sharp tips. Bring to a boil 2 cups of water, to which you have added

Serves two:
2 large artichokes
sea salt
dash of cider vinegar
bunch of basil
1 soft avocado
2 tbsp lemon juice
1 tsp black cumin oil
white pepper

a pinch of salt and the vinegar. Cook the artichokes for about 30 minutes, until you can easily pull out a leaf. Reserve the cooking liquid.

Wash and shake dry the basil, and remove the leaves from the stalks. Halve the avocado, and remove the stone. Purée the flesh, a little of the cooking liquid, and some lemon juice, and add the oil, salt, and pepper. Season the dip with salt and pepper, and serve as an accompaniment to the warm or cooled artichokes.

Versatile artichokes

Artichokes contain the bitter cynarine, which stimulates the liver and thereby cleanses the blood. It also stimulates cell renewal – and that's good for the skin. Beta-carotene and vitamin E aid this effect. You can add honey to the cooking liquid, then refrigerate it and serve as an aperitif.

PER PORTION:

180 kcal

5 g protein

14 g fat

11 g carbohydrate

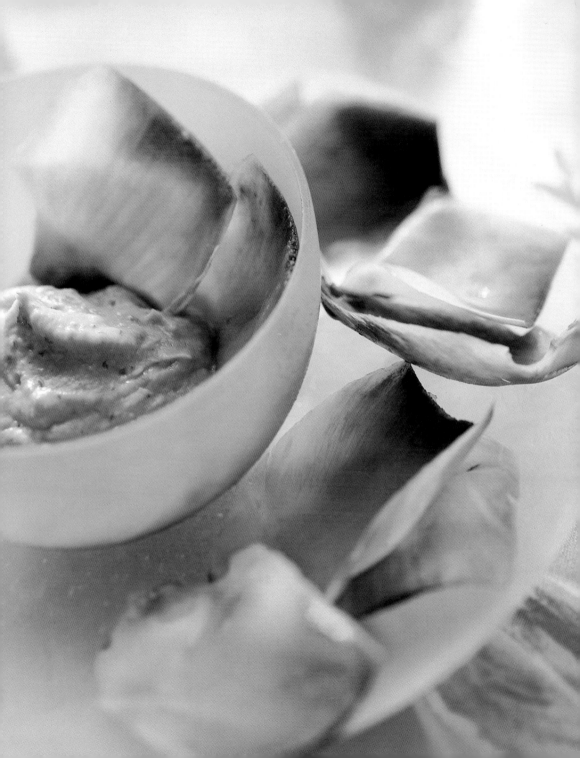

Grapefruit and
Raw Carrot Salad
with red lentils and sea vegetables

Serves two:

15 g/¹/₂ oz sea vegetables
(eg 2 tbsp arame)
300 ml (12 fl oz) water
150 g (5 oz) red lentils
sea salt
1 tsp powdered ginger
200 g (7 oz) young carrots
200 g (7 oz) spinach
1 small onion
1 pink grapefruit
3 tbsp wheatgerm oil
1 tsp mustard powder
black pepper

Soak the sea vegetables in the water for 10 minutes. Then place in a saucepan with the red lentils, salt, and powdered ginger. Cover with a lid and cook over a low heat for about 10 minutes. Do not cook for any longer, as the sea vegetables would absorb too much liquid.

Meanwhile, wash and peel the carrots, and grate coarsely. Wash and pick over the spinach, remove any coarse stalks, and cut the leaves into strips. Peel and finely chop the onion. Halve the grapefruit and use a spoon to scoop out the flesh. Squeeze the juice from the grapefruit halves. Add the juice, the grapefruit pieces, wheatgerm oil, and mustard powder to the lentil and sea vegetables mixture, and carefully stir in the grated carrot and spinach strips. Season well with salt and pepper, and serve warm immediately, accompanied by rice.

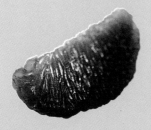

Grapefruit
Just one grapefruit provides an adult's daily vitamin C requirement. It also stimulates the circulatory system.

PER PORTION:

440 kcal

22 g protein

17 g fat

51 g carbohydrate

power

Broccoli and

with probiotic yogurt and lots of vitamin E

Sauerkraut Salad

Wash the broccoli florets and drain in a strainer. Chop them a little, then purée, adding a little water. Drain the sweetcorn in a strainer. Coarsely chop the sauerkraut with a knife, then add to the sweetcorn and puréed broccoli. Coarsely chop the sunflower seeds. Peel and finely chop the garlic. To make the dressing, place the sunflower seeds, garlic, yogurt, oil, and vinegar in a bowl, and mix well. Season to taste with salt, pepper, thyme, and ginger. Pour the dressing over the vegetables. Arrange the salad on plates, and serve with bread or boiled new potatoes.

Serves two:

150 g (5 oz) broccoli florets

1–2 tbsp water

150 g (5 oz) sweetcorn (small can)

200 g (7 oz) fresh sauerkraut

2 tbsp sunflower seeds

1 garlic clove

150 g (5 fl oz) probiotic yogurt

2 tbsp nut oil

1–2 tbsp cider vinegar

sea salt

black pepper

1 tsp thyme leaves

$^1/_2$ tsp powdered ginger

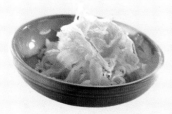

Sauerkraut

Sauerkraut contains plenty of lactic acid, potassium, calcium, and iodine, as well as vitamin C. It aids digestion and strengthens tissues. Fresh sauerkraut from a delicatessen is especially effective.

PER PORTION:

355 kcal

11 g protein

23 g fat

31 g carbohydrate

power

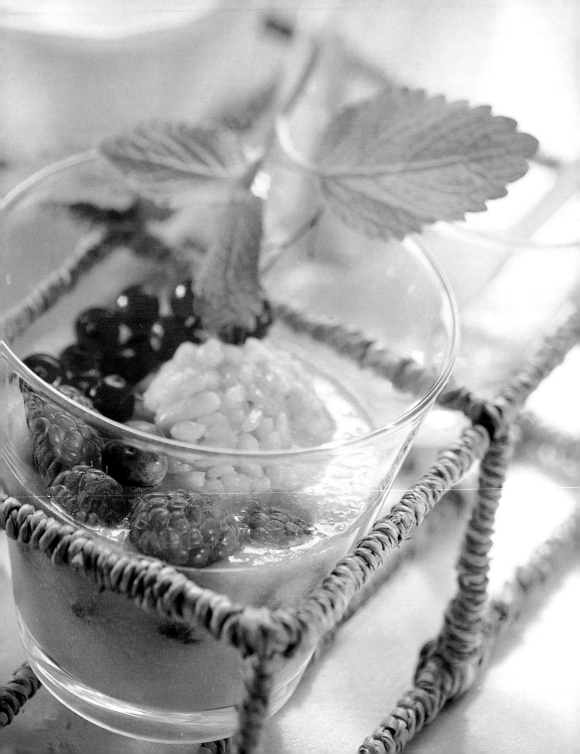

Melon
with vitamin risotto
Fruit Purée

Heat the oil in a pan over a low heat. Add the pudding rice and the pine kernels, and simmer gently until the rice becomes translucent. Then pour over half of the juice, and simmer gently, stirring continuously, until the rice starts to become grainy. Then add the remaining juice, and bring to a boil again briefly. Place on one side, cover with a lid, and leave for 4 hours or overnight, until completely cool. Peel and seed the melon. Purée the flesh, adding the honey. Add the berries. Place the fruit purée in deep bowls. Top with a scoop of the cooked rice and serve.

Serves two:

1 tsp wheatgerm oil

80 g (3 oz) pudding rice

2 tbsp pine kernels

300 ml (12 fl oz) apple/orange/grape juice

$^1/_2$ charentais melon (350 g/12 oz flesh)

1 tbsp honey

1 cup berries (to taste)

Multi-vitamin fruit juices

Some fruit juices contain added pro-vitamin A, vitamins C and E, and often omega-3 fatty acids. They are one of the most probiotic (health-promoting) foods, and their primary task is cell protection.

PER PORTION:

425 kcal

7 g protein

6 g fat

84 g carbohydrate

Fruit Salad
and toasted buckwheat
with Grapes

Serves two: · 200 g (7 oz) seedless grapes · 1 apple · 1 orange · 2 tbsp raisins · 100 ml (4 fl oz) apple/orange/grape juice · 50 g (2 oz) buckwheat · 2 tbsp sesame seeds

Wash the fruit. Remove the stalks from the grapes. Cut the apple into eight pieces, remove the seeds, and cut each slice in half widthwise. Peel the orange, divide into segments, and cut each segment into three. Rinse the raisins in hot water, and mix with the fruit and juice. Dry-fry the buckwheat and sesame seeds in a nonstick pan until you can smell them. Cool, then sprinkle over the fruit salad.

PER PORTION: 295 kcal • 6 g protein • 5 g fat • 60 g carbohydrate

Orange and
with high-vitamin C rosehip syrup
Carrot Quark

Serves two: · 2 young carrots · 1 orange · 1 tbsp rosehip syrup, sweetened · 1 tbsp honey · 250 g (9 oz) quark (20% fat) · 20 g ($^3/_4$ oz) flaked almonds

Wash, peel, and finely grate the carrots. Peel the orange and cut into slices, then cut each slice into eight. Combine the rosehip pulp with the honey. Gradually add to the quark. Stir in the grated carrot, orange pieces with juice, and the almonds.

PER PORTION: 335 kcal • 17 g protein • 12 g fat • 41 g carbohydrate

Choco
with dried dates
Risotto

Wash the dates, remove the skin and stones, and chop into small pieces.

Place the rice in a saucepan and warm gently over a low heat, then pour over the milk. Add the chopped dates, cocoa powder, and cane sugar.

Cover with a lid and simmer gently over a low heat for about 50 minutes, stirring occasionally. Leave the rice to cool. Alternatively, bring the rice to a boil, then wrap the pan of rice in cloths and leave for 3–4 hours.

Beat the cream until stiff. Gently combine with the rice and serve immediately.

Serves two:
100 g (4 oz) dried dates
100 g (4 oz) risotto rice
500 ml (20 fl oz) milk (semi-skimmed)
1 tbsp cocoa powder
2 tbsp cane sugar
100 ml (4 fl oz) whipping cream

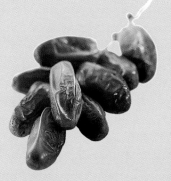

Dates

These dried fruits contain plenty of iron and potassium. Because they are naturally sweet, they are an ideal substitute for sugar. They are high in fibre, which gently stimulates the digestion. If you do not have such a sweet tooth, look for previously frozen dates that are sold all year round as fresh.

Per Portion:

560 kcal

10 g protein

18 g fat

87 g carbohydrate

Bean and
with vitamin-packed sea vegetables
Shrimp Salad

Serves two:

15 g/½ oz sea vegetables
(eg 2 tbsp arame)

300 g (10 oz) green beans

1 onion

1 tbsp olive oil

sea salt and black pepper

1 tsp thyme leaves

200 g (7 oz) tomatoes

10 black olives

200 g (7 oz) shrimps

2–3 tbsp cider vinegar

Soak the sea vegetables in 300 ml (12 fl oz) water. Meanwhile, wash and trim the beans, and remove any strings. Peel, halve, and finely chop the onion. Heat the oil, and glaze the diced onion and beans over medium heat. Add the sea vegetables with the water used for soaking. Season the vegetables with salt and pepper. Add the thyme and simmer everything gently for about 15 minutes. Leave to cool.

Wash the tomatoes, remove the cores, and cut into thin segments. Remove the pits from the olives, and cut into thin slices.

Drain the shrimps and add to the beans with the tomatoes and olives. Season to taste with cider vinegar.

Olives & oil – a healthy duo

Olives are good for the circulation, and stabilize blood pressure. They contain lactic acid, which is full of unsaturated fatty acids. The most important ingredient is squalene, which keeps the skin healthy and smooth, and stimulates the immune system.

PER PORTION:

225 kcal

23 g protein

9 g fat

14 g carbohydrate

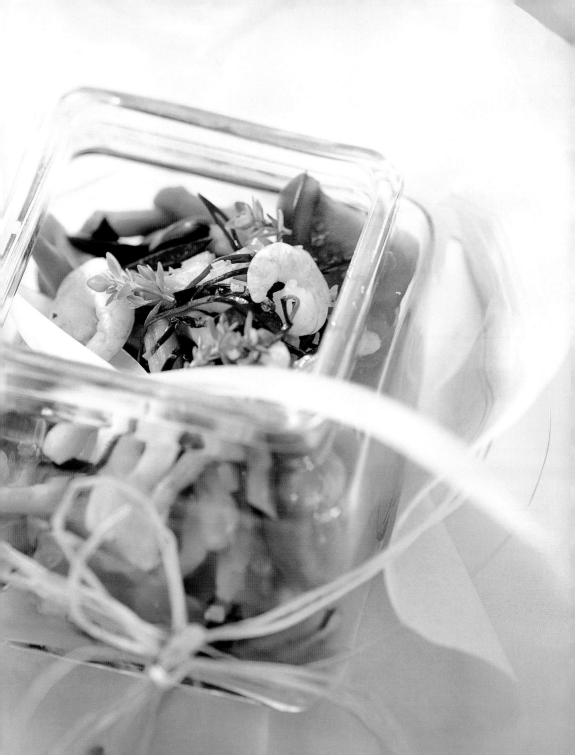

Cabbage Salad

sweet and sour with sauerkraut and nuts

with Apples

Wash the cabbage and apples. Cut the cabbage into quarters, remove the core, and finely slice the cabbage pieces. Dry the apples and grate them coarsely without peeling them. In a bowl, combine the sliced cabbage with the grated apple. Stir the sauerkraut and lemon juice into the apple and cabbage mixture. Season well with salt and pepper. Leave to stand for about 1 hour.

Meanwhile, wash the dill, remove the tips from the stalks, and chop. Coarsely chop the walnuts. To make the dressing, stir together the sour cream, dill, walnuts, aniseed, and wheatgerm oil, and season with salt and pepper. Stir the dressing into the salad, seasoning again if necessary.

Serves two:
200 g (7 oz) white cabbage
2 apples
125 ml (4½ fl oz) sauerkraut juice
2–3 tbsp lemon juice
sea salt
pepper
bunch of dill
60 g (2 oz) walnuts
150 ml (6 fl oz) sour cream (10% fat)
½ tsp aniseed
1 tbsp wheatgerm oil

Not quite so tough

In fall and winter, when cabbages are firmer and a little harder to digest, heat the sauerkraut and lemon juices before pouring them over the cabbage. Leave to stand for about 1 hour until cool. Do not add the grated apple until the cabbage has cooled.

Per Portion:

425 kcal

9 g protein

32 g fat

24 g carbohydrate

Bulgur Salad
contains lots of lactic acid and fermented wheat liquid
with Garlic

Peel the garlic and cut into thin slices. Pour the fermented wheat liquid into a pan, then add the garlic and bring to a boil. Pour over the bulgur wheat, season with salt and pepper, and simmer gently for about 5 minutes over a low heat. Leave to cool.

Meanwhile, halve the bell pepper, and remove the stalk, seeds, and pith. Wash, cut lengthwise into strips, then dice the strips. Wash and shake dry the parsley. Pull the tips from the stalks, and coarsely chop. Stir the bell pepper, parsley, olives, borage oil, and capers into the bulgur.

Finely crumble the feta cheese and sprinkle over the bulgur mixture. Season well with salt and pepper, adding a little more fermented wheat liquid if necessary. Arrange on plates and serve.

Serves two:

4 garlic cloves

250 ml (10 fl oz) fermented wheat liquid

120 g (4¹/₂ oz) bulgur (cracked wheat)

sea salt

black pepper

1 red bell pepper (capsicum)

2 bunches Italian parsley

1 tbsp olive oil

1 tsp borage (star flower) oil

2 tbsp capers

120 g (4¹/₂ oz) feta cheese

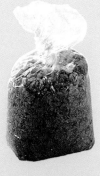

Bulgur

Bulgur is coarsely broken wheat that can be cooked like parboiled rice. You will find it in most health-food stores and supermarkets. It contains large amounts of protein and B-complex vitamins.

PER PORTION:

470 kcal

23 g protein

19 g fat

55 g carbohydrate

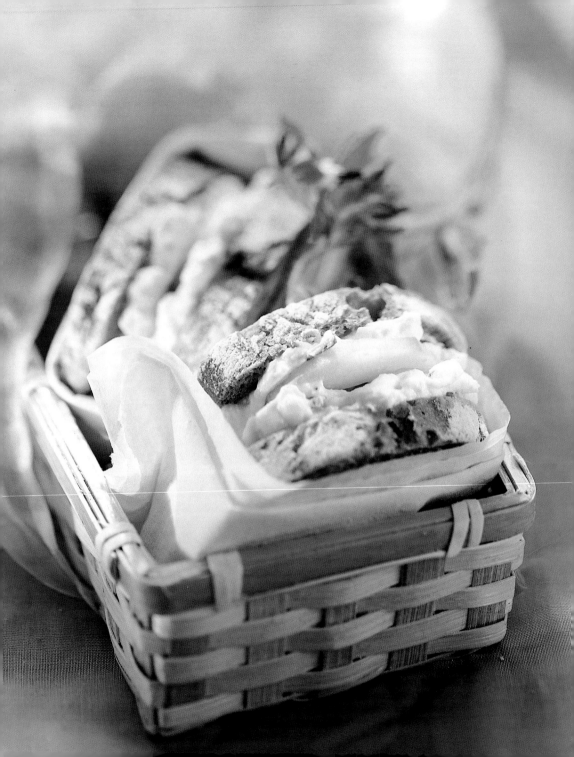

Goat's Cheese
with borage oil and leaves
Sandwich

Peel and halve the cucumber, and scoop out the seeds with a spoon. Grate half the cucumber, and cut the other piece into fairly thin slices. Peel and finely chop the onion. Wash and shake dry the borage leaves, then finely chop.

Combine with borage oil with the onion, borage leaves, grated cucumber, and goat's cheese.

Divide the cheese between the two slices of bread, and top with the sliced cucumber, pressing down slightly. Season with salt and pepper, sprinkle with the sunflower seeds, and serve. Top with a second slice of bread if you want to use the sandwiches in a packed lunch.

Serves two:
$^1/_2$ cucumber
1 small onion
few borage leaves
2 tbsp borage (star flower) oil
120 g (4$^1/_2$ oz) fresh goat's cheese
sea salt
pepper
2 slices wholewheat bread
1 tbsp sunflower seeds

Easy to digest

Goat's cheese contains less cholesterol than other types of cheese. It also contains lots of vitamin A, which keeps the skin smooth and the eyes shining. It is widely available.

PER PORTION:

305 kcal

17 g protein

19 g fat

16 g carbohydrate

Salmon and Cress
secret weapon for fighting skin irritations
Sandwich

Serves two: · 2 bread rolls with grains · 1 punnet of cress · 4 tbsp crème fraîche · 1 tsp borage (star flower) oil · sea salt · black pepper · 1 tsp lemon juice · 4 slices of smoked salmon

Cut the bread rolls in half. Rinse the cress under cold running water, and snip off the leaves, reserving some for garnish. Combine the remaining cress with the crème fraîche, borage oil, salt, pepper, and lemon juice, and spread on the halved bread rolls. Top with the smoked salmon slices, and garnish with the cress.

PER PORTION: 330 kcal •22 g protein • 17 g fat • 22 g carbohydrate

Dry-cured Beef
with fresh sauerkraut and horseradish
Sandwich

Serves two: · 2 tbsp horseradish · 4 tbsp cottage cheese · 1 tsp pumpkin seed oil · 1 tbsp chopped pumpkin seeds · 2 slices of bread with linseeds · black pepper · 50 g ($1^3/_4$ oz) sauerkraut · 6 slices of dry-cured beef

Combine the horseradish with the cottage cheese, oil, and pumpkin seeds. Spread over the bread, and grate over some pepper. Chop the sauerkraut and sprinkle over the cheese mixture. Fold the slices of meat in half and arrange decoratively on top.

PER PORTION: 230 kcal •18 g protein • 9 g fat • 17 g carbohydrate

Tuna and Egg
with capers and olive oil
Sandwich

Serves two: · 1 can of tuna fish in brine (160 g/5¹/₂ oz meat) · 3 tbsp olive oil · 1 hard-boiled egg · 1 tbsp lemon juice · 2 tbsp capers · pepper · Worcestershire sauce · 2 wholewheat bread rolls · 2–3 radicchio leaves

Drain the tuna fish. Purée with the olive oil, egg yolk, and lemon juice, using a hand-held blender. Season to taste with the capers, pepper, and Worcestershire sauce. Halve the rolls, and spread with the paste. Wash and pat dry the radicchio leaves, cut into strips, and arrange on the rolls. Chop the egg white and sprinkle over.

PER PORTION: 515 kcal •27 g protein • 33 g fat • 28 g carbohydrate

Black Pesto
with fresh rye bread and basil
Sandwich

Serves two: · 2 slices of rye bread · 2 tsp pesto (ready made) · 1 tbsp sesame seeds · ¹/₂ bunch of basil · 150 g (5 oz) mozzarella · 8 cherry tomatoes

Spread the bread with the pesto, and sprinkle over the sesame seeds. Wash and shake dry the basil, then remove the leaves and place on the bread. Drain the mozzarella, cut into slices, and place on the bread. Wash and halve the tomatoes, remove the stalks, and arrange on the mozzarella. Grate over some pepper.

PER PORTION: 275 kcal •19 g protein • 16 g fat • 13 g carbohydrate

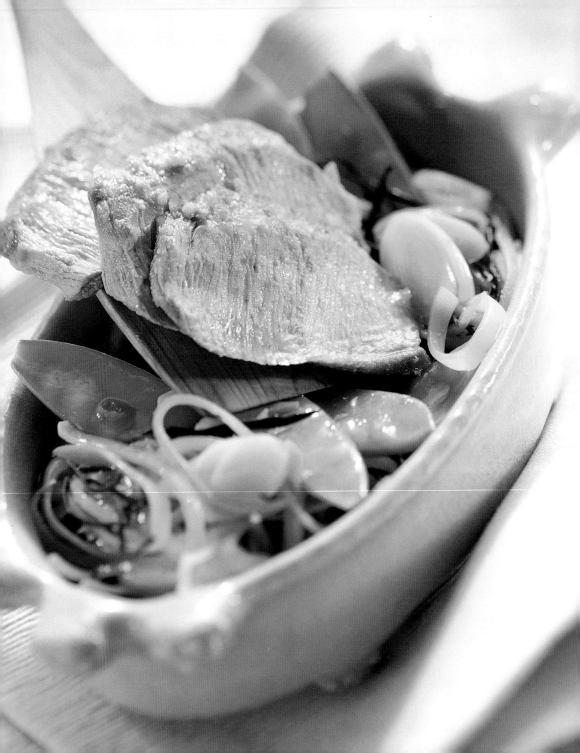

Lamb Noisettes

stimulating and full of minerals

with Vegetables

Soak the sea vegetables in 125 ml (4 fl oz) water for about 10 minutes.

Wash and pat dry the meat. Peel and finely chop the ginger, and combine

with the mustard powder, soy sauce, lemon
juice, and 2 tbsp of water. Brush over the meat.
Wash and trim the other vegetables. Halve the
leek lengthwise and slice into fine rings. Peel
the carrots and cut into fine strips. Break the
ends off the sugar snap peas or beans, and
remove any strings.

Drain the sea vegetables. Heat the dripping in a
nonstick pan, and brown the meat on both
sides. Add the vegetables and the sea
vegetables. Season and stir-fry for about 5–7
minutes. Season with soy sauce and sesame oil.
Serve with potatoes, wild rice, or millet.

Serves two:

15 g/¹/₂ oz sea vegetables (eg 2 tbsp arame)

300 g (10 oz) lamb noisettes

piece of ginger

1 tsp mustard powder

1 tbsp soy sauce

2 tbsp lemon juice

1 leek

200 g (7 oz) carrots

150 g (5 oz) sugar snap peas or beans

1 tsp dripping

sea salt

pepper

1 tbsp sesame oil

PER PORTION: 330 kcal • 50 g protein • 15 g fat • 43 g carbohydrate

Mussel

with feta and chilli

Rosti

Wash the potatoes, and parboil them in a little salted water for about 10 minutes. Rinse under cold water, then peel. Cool slightly before grating coarsely. Meanwhile, wash and trim the spring onion and chilli. Cut the spring onion into thin rings and finely chop the chilli. Peel and finely chop the garlic, finely dice the tomatoes, and drain the mussels. Crumble the feta cheese and combine with the grated potato, spring onion, chilli, garlic, tomatoes, and mussels. Season well with salt, pepper, and star anise.

Heat 1–2 tbsp olive oil in a nonstick frying pan, and spread the mixture over the base. Press down firmly, cover with a lid, and fry over a low heat for about 7 minutes, until golden. Turn, and fry the other side until golden, adding a little oil if necessary. Serve with a tomato salad.

Serves two:
400 g (14 oz) floury potatoes
sea salt
1 spring onion
1 chilli pod
1 garlic clove
3 sun-dried tomatoes
250 g (8 oz) jar of mussels
50 g (1³/₄ oz) feta cheese
black pepper
star anise
olive oil for frying

Chilli

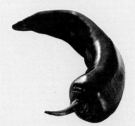

The pods are incredibly hot, especially the white pith and the seeds. The spiciness stimulates the digestion and circulation, and helps to prevent infection. Avoid contact with the skin, and especially the nose and eyes: chilli burns.

PER PORTION:

560 kcal

36 g protein

14 g fat

82 g carbohydrate

Mashed
with pickled herring and healthy whey
Potatoes

Soak the pickled fish in water for at least 1–2 hours. Wash the potatoes, and boil in a little lightly salted water for about 20 minutes. Peel and set aside.

Meanwhile, wash and shake dry the chives, then chop finely. Wash the radishes, keeping 4 of them and a few of the tender leaves for garnish. Trim and dice the remainder.

In a pan, heat the potatoes with the whey and rapeseed oil over a medium heat, then mash the potatoes coarsely with a masher. Add the chives and the diced radishes, then season with salt and pepper, and heat through.

Remove the fish from the water, pat dry, and arrange on plates with the reserved radishes and potatoes. Sprinkle over the chopped radish leaves, and serve.

Serves two:
4 matjes herring fillets
400 g (14 oz) floury potatoes
sea salt
bunch of chives
bunch of radishes
125 ml (4¹/₂ fl oz) whey
1 tbsp rapeseed oil
white pepper

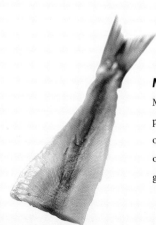

Matjes herring

Matjes is pre-adolescent herring. It is particularly delicate, and contains plenty of oil. Since herring contains plenty of omega-3 fatty acids, matjes are especially good for the skin and general wellbeing.

PER PORTION:

625 kcal

31 g protein

44 g fat

27 g carbohydrate

Carrot and
Millet Spaghetti

lots of vitamins and minerals

Serves two:
250 g (9 oz) fresh, green-topped carrots
1 onion
1 garlic clove
1 tbsp sesame oil
2 tbsp sesame seeds
sea salt
pepper
star anise
pinch of saffron powder
100 ml (4 fl oz) orange juice
250 g (9 oz) millet spaghetti

Wash the carrots and a handful of the green tops. Trim and peel the carrots, and slice into long strips with a vegetable peeler. Peel and finely chop the onion and the garlic. Heat the sesame oil and brown the sesame seeds. Add the onion and the garlic, and sauté over a medium heat until translucent.

Add the carrot strips and season with salt, pepper, and star anise. Cover with a lid and simmer gently over a low heat for 1–2 minutes. Combine the saffron powder with the orange juice. Once the carrots are just beginning to catch, pour over the juice and the green tops, and stir. Simmer gently for another 2–3 minutes over a low heat until the carrots are ready.

Meanwhile, cook the pasta in plenty of boiling salted water until *al dente*. Drain in a strainer and rinse in cold water. Drain, and combine with the cooked carrots. Arrange on plates and serve immediately.

PER PORTION: 560 kcal • 22 g protein • 11 g fat • 93 g carbohydrate

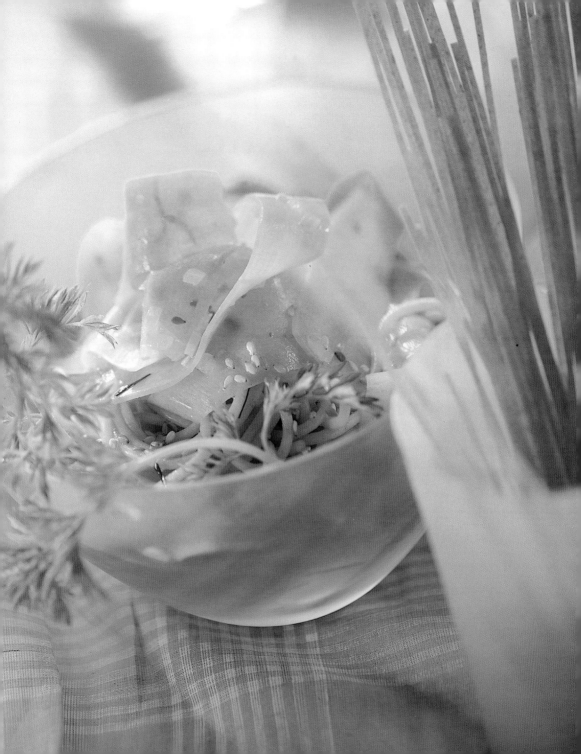

Blue Cheese and
with sea vegetables and spaghetti mix
Tomato Sauce

Soak the sea vegetables in 250 ml (10 fl oz) water for about 5 minutes. Meanwhile, wash and slit the tomatoes. Dip in boiling water, then skin, remove the stalks, and purée. Peel and finely chop the onion. To make the sauce, heat 1 tbsp of oil and sauté the onion gently over a medium heat. Add the puréed tomato and tomato paste, and simmer briefly over a low heat. Bring plenty of salted water to a boil. Drain the sea vegetables and boil, with the spaghetti, until *al dente*. Drain, rinse under cold water, then drain again. Combine the sea vegetables and spaghetti with the lemon juice and 1 tbsp of oil. Remove the rind from the cheese, crumble, and dissolve in the tomato sauce. Season well with soy sauce, pepper and paprika. Add a little water to the sauce if it is too thick. Arrange on plates and serve.

Serves two:

15 g/¹/₂ oz sea vegetables
(eg 2 tbsp arame)
500 g (1 lb 2 oz) ripe tomatoes
1 onion
2 tbsp wheatgerm oil
2 tbsp tomato paste
sea salt
200 g (7 oz) millet spaghetti
1–2 tbsp lemon juice
150 g (5 oz) blue cheese
soy sauce
pepper
mild ground paprika

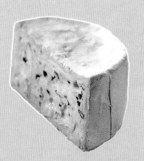

Blue cheese

This is injected with blue cheese cultures and then left to mature until it has developed the characteristic blue-green veins. It is full of protein, easy to digest, and its enzymes have a beneficial effect on intestinal flora and the digestion in general.

PER PORTION:

810 kcal

33 g protein

43 g fat

73 g carbohydrate

power

Green
with fresh asparagus and leaf spinach
Ratatouille

Wash the cucumber, and cut in half lengthwise. Remove the seeds, and cut into 1 cm (¹/₂ in) slices. Wash and trim the asparagus, peel carefully, and cut into 2–3 cm (³/₄–1 in) pieces. Trim and pick over the rocket, then wash, shake dry, and chop finely. Wash and pick over the spinach, break off any coarse stalks, and chop roughly. Peel and finely chop the onion and garlic. Heat the oil and sauté the onion and garlic over a medium heat. Add the asparagus and the cucumber. Season with salt, pepper, and nutmeg, and cover with a lid. Simmer gently for about 10 minutes over a low heat. Add the spinach and the rocket, season with salt and pepper, and simmer for another 3 minutes. Add more seasoning if necessary. Divide the ratatouille between plates, drizzle over some borage oil, and grate over a little Parmesan.

Serves two:

1 cucumber
250 g (9 oz) asparagus
bunch of rocket
250 g (9 oz) fresh spinach leaves
1 onion
1 garlic clove
1 tbsp olive oil
sea salt and pepper
nutmeg
2 tsp borage (star flower) oil
50 g (1³/₄ oz) Parmesan, whole

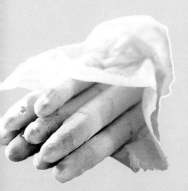

Asparagus

Asparagus contains aspartic acid and potassium, which stimulate the kidneys and are diuretic. It is also extremely low in calories, and is excellent for a weight-reducing diet if it is also prepared with few calories. Although its benefits are not dependent on the variety, green asparagus contains more vitamins.

PER PORTION:

215 kcal

17 g protein

10 g fat

13 g carbohydrate

power

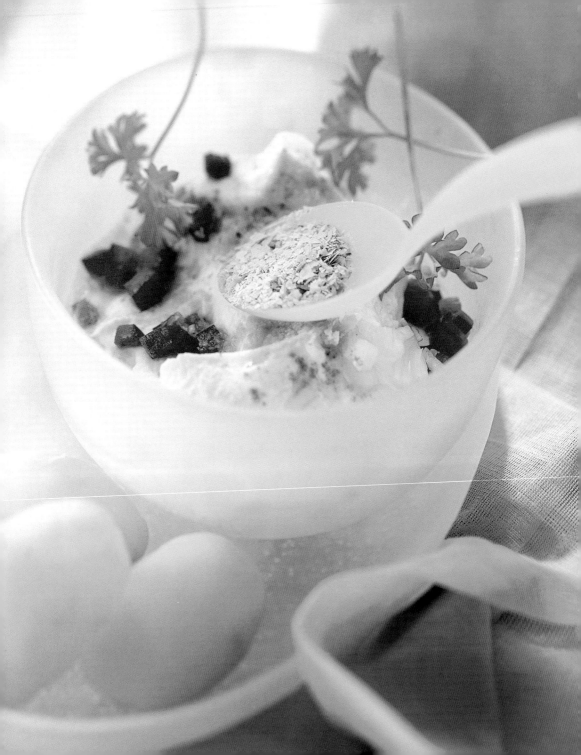

Boiled New Potatoes

ideal for nerves and stomach

with Power Quark

Wash the potatoes. Cover with a lid and boil in a little salted water for about 20 minutes. Meanwhile, halve the bell pepper, and remove the stalks, seeds, and pith. Wash, then chop into small dice. Peel and finely chop the shallot and the garlic. Wash and pat dry the parsley, remove the leaves from the stalks, and finely chop.

Place the quark in a bowl and combine with the parsley, wheatgerm, yeast flakes, linseed oil, chilli pepper or tabasco, and enough mineral water to make a smooth cream. Add the chopped bell pepper, the diced shallot, and the garlic. Season well, and serve with the potatoes.

Serves two:
500 g (1 lb 2 oz) new potatoes
sea salt
1 small, red bell pepper (capsicum)
1 shallot
1 garlic clove
bunch of parsley
250 g (9 oz) low-fat quark
1 tbsp wheatgerm
1 tbsp yeast flakes
1 tbsp linseed (flax) oil
chilli pepper or tabasco
100 ml (4 fl oz) mineral water

Potatoes – getting down to the roots

Potatoes contain plenty of valuable plant protein and vitamin C, and are thus an important basic food. The raw juice, which is available from health-food stores, is excellent for the stomach, and ideal for over-acidity. Served with quark, they are at least as nutritious as a small steak, and the fibre they contain stimulates the digestion. Never eat uncooked potatoes.

PER PORTION:

335 kcal

25 g protein

9 g fat

41 g carbohydrate

Turkey Breast
mildly spicy and tender
with Chicory

Serves two:

200 g (7 oz) turkey breast fillet

sea salt and pepper

mild ground paprika

2 small heads of chicory
(300 g/10 oz)

1 tsp clarified butter

250 g (9 oz) diced tomatoes
(canned)

piece of ginger

1 garlic clove

100 g (4 oz) bean sprouts

1 tbsp sesame oil

100 g (4 oz) mozzarella

Cut the turkey breast against the grain into 1 cm (½ in) slices. Season with salt, pepper, and paprika. Wash and trim the chicory, and halve lengthwise. Melt the butter in a pot and sauté the chicory until just brown at the edges. Add the turkey meat and brown on all sides. Add the tomatoes and season with salt and pepper. Cover with a lid and simmer gently for 5 minutes over a low heat.

Meanwhile, peel the ginger and the garlic, and grate into thin slices. Add to the meat with the bean sprouts and oil. Drain the mozzarella, cut into slices, and place on the chicory. Simmer gently over a low heat until the cheese has melted. Arrange on plates and serve with a baguette.

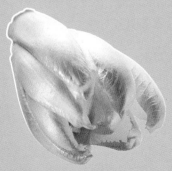

Chicory

Its bitter constituents stimulate the stomach, spleen, liver, and gall bladder – it is a veritable "spa food". Its constituents - including special carbohydrates known as fos (fructooligosaccharides) - influence intestinal health and help regenerate the membranes and flora of the intestine.

PER PORTION:

350 kcal

40 g protein

17 g fat

10 g carbohydrate

power

Beef Chilli

spicy and wonderfully stimulating

with Avocado

To make the marinade, combine the lemon juice, salt, pepper, ground paprika, and star anise. Cut the meat into fine strips against the grain, and place in the marinade. Slit open the chilli pepper and remove the seeds. Wash, then finely chop. Halve the bell pepper, remove the stalk, seeds, and pith, and chop coarsely. Peel and finely chop the garlic and the onions. Drain the meat. Heat the oil and brown the meat on all sides. Add the chilli, paprika, onions, and garlic, and stir-fry for another 5 minutes. Wash and shake dry the parsley, remove the stalks, and chop the florets. Halve the avocado, remove the pit, and chop. Combine the avocado, olives, parsley, and marinade, then heat and season. Serve with boiled millet, creamed corn, or bread.

Serves two:
3 tbsp lemon juice
sea salt and pepper
pinch of hot ground paprika
$^{1}/_{2}$ tsp star anise
200 g (7 oz) thinly sliced beef steak
1 chilli pepper
1 green bell pepper (capsicum)
2 garlic cloves
2 onions
1–2 tbsp olive oil
bunch of Italian parsley
1 avocado
10 black olives

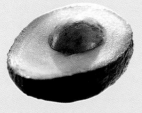

Avocado

This is a tonic for the stomach, nerves, skin, and hair – provided it is ripe and as soft as butter. It contains 30% valuable plant fats, and lots of B-complex vitamins. Mashed with a few drops of lemon juice, salt, and pepper, it makes an ideal spread.

PER PORTION:

390 kcal

26 g protein

26 g fat

17 g carbohydrate

Salmon
with feta and fennel seeds
on Fennel

Wash and part dry the fillets. Sprinkle with cider vinegar, then season with salt and pepper. Wash and trim the fennel, and cut into thin slices. Reserve a little of the green. Wash and peel the potatoes, and cut into 1 cm (1\2 in) cubes. Wash and shake dry the dill, remove the tips, and combine with the fennel green.

Serves two:
2 small salmon fillets (each 200 g/7 oz)
2 tbsp cider vinegar
sea salt and pepper
1 small head of fennel
400 g (14 oz) potatoes
bunch of dill
1 tbsp wheatgerm
1 tbsp fennel seeds
100 g (4 oz) feta cheese

Heat the oil and braise the fennel. Add the diced potatoes, and season with salt and pepper. Pour over 150 ml (5 fl oz) water, sprinkle over the fennel seeds, and simmer for 5 minutes.

Sprinkle the dill and fennel mix over the fish, and place the fish on the fennel and potato mixture. Crumble over the feta, and simmer everything gently for another 15 minutes.

Cider vinegar – modern medicine

There's a good reason why cider vinegar is currently so popular: it fights putrefactive bacteria in the intestine, kills germs, aids detoxification, and improves digestion. It is also slightly milder than wine vinegar, so is excellent in the kitchen.

PER PORTION:

525 kcal

55g protein

20 g fat

28 g carbohydrate

power

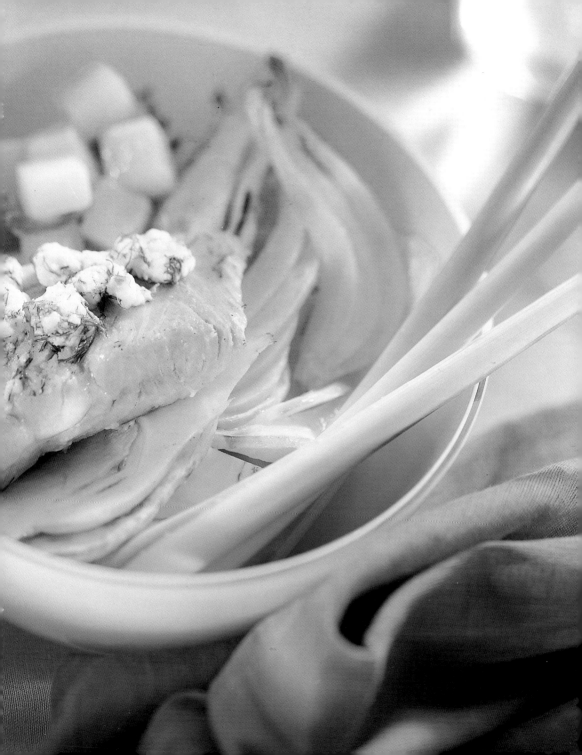

Fried

sour-sweet with coconut and pineapple

Seafood Rice

Heat the rice in a pan, then add 200 ml (8 fl oz) water and the salt, and bring to a boil. Cover with a lid and simmer gently for 20 minutes. Wash, trim, and peel the carrots, and cut into slices. Remove the stalk, seeds, and pith from the bell pepper, then wash and dice. Trim the spring onion and slice into thin rings. Scoop the flesh from the coconut shell, and chop the flesh.

Peel the ginger and grate into thin slices. Peel and halve the baby pineapple, remove the core, and chop the flesh.

Heat the oil in a large frying pan or wok. Fry the carrots and spring onion, then gradually add the coconut, ginger, and bean sprouts, stirring continuously. Add the rice, pineapple, and the shrimp or prawns, and fry. Season with soy sauce and serve immediately.

Serves two:
120 g (4¹/₂ oz) wholewheat Basmati rice
1 tsp sea salt
2 fresh carrots (150 g/5 oz)
¹/₂ red bell pepper (capsicum)
1 spring onion
¹/₂ small coconut (or 3 tbsp grated)
small piece of ginger
1 baby pineapple
1–2 tbsp rapeseed oil
1 cup bean sprouts (100 g/4 oz)
150 g (5 oz) shrimps or prawns
soy sauce

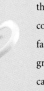

Soybeans

Sprouting improves the constituents of the soybean: it increases the vitamin content, breaks down protein, makes the fat more digestible, and encourages the growth of enzymes. By contrast, the calorie content drops after sprouting.

PER PORTION:

600 kcal

26 g protein

24 g fat

70 g carbohydrate

power

Radicchio and
with plums and black Puy lentils
Fish Stew

Wash and pat dry the fish fillets, then sprinkle over the cider vinegar and season with salt. Trim the leek and slit open lengthwise. Wash and cut into thin slices. Cut the prunes lengthwise into quarters. Heat the oil in a frying pan and glaze the leek over medium heat. Pour over the potato juice, then add salt, the bay leaf, peppercorns, cloves, prunes, and lentils. Cover with a lid and simmer gently over a low heat for about 8 minutes.

Meanwhile, trim and wash the radicchio, and cut the leaves into strips. Add the radicchio and the fish, with the marinade, to the lentils, and simmer gently for another 3–4 minutes over a low heat.

Season with honey and salt. Arrange on plates and serve with a baguette.

Note: If potato juice is unavailable, use the water from boiled potatoes.

Serves two:
300 g (10 oz) fish fillets
3 tbsp cider vinegar
sea salt
1 leek
10 prunes
1 tbsp nut oil
500 ml (20 fl oz) potato juice
(from a health-food store)
1 bay leaf
3 peppercorns
2 cloves
100 g (4 oz) black lentils
1 radicchio (150 g/5 oz)
1 tsp honey

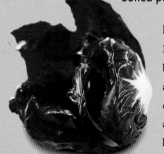

Radicchio

It tastes – and works – like bitters. Its bitter constituents stimulate the digestion and at the same time are soothing and cleanse the blood. It is related to chicory and is just as calming. Unfortunately, it loses its lovely red colour when cooked.

PER PORTION:

525 kcal

43 g protein

9 g fat

65 g carbohydrate

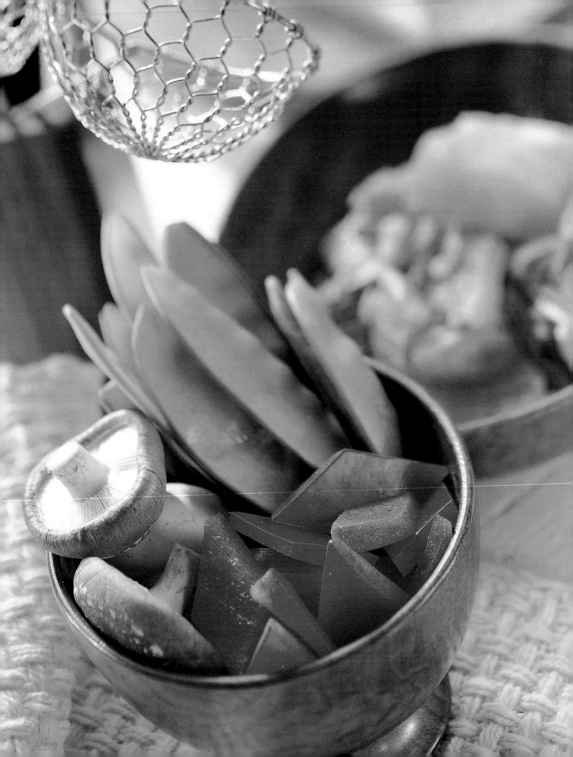

Chinese
excellent with fresh salmon trout
Fondue

Wash and pat dry the fish, and cut crosswise into 3 cm (1 1\4 in) strips. Cut each strip into 4 cm (1 1\2 in) pieces. Peel and finely chop the ginger. Trim, wash, and thinly slice the spring onion. Squeeze the juice from the lime and reserve 1 teaspoon of the juice. Mix the remaining juice with the ginger and sliced spring onion. Sprinkle over the fish, then season with salt and pepper, and put in the refrigerator.

Wash and trim the sugar snap peas, and slice diagonally. Brush the mushrooms. Wash and halve the bell pepper, and remove the stalk, seeds, and pith, then slice diagonally. Put the sugar snap peas, mushrooms, and bell pepper in the refrigerator. Heat the stock with the remaining lime juice and the lemon grass. Light the fondue burner. Pour the stock into the fondue pot, and place over the burner. Put the fish and the vegetables in fondue baskets, and cook in the stock. Serve with soy sauce, rice, and dips.

Serves two:
400 g (14 oz) Norwegian salmon trout, filleted
piece of ginger
1 spring onion
1 lime
sea salt
pepper
200 g (7 oz) sugar snap peas
200 g (7 oz) button or shiitake mushrooms
1 red bell pepper (capsicum)
1.5 litres (2¹/₂ pints) chicken stock (granules or cube)
2–3 stalks of lemon grass

PER PORTION: 315 kcal • 65 g protein • 10 g fat• 52 g carbohydrate

Eggplant and Prawns

grilled on a hot griddle

Wash the eggplant, remove the stalk, and cut diagonally into thin slices. Salt the slices, stack to make two towers, and cover with a chopping board. Wash the prawns.

Serves two:
1 small eggplant (200 g/7 oz)
sea salt
8 king prawns
1 chilli pepper
1 spring onion
1 garlic clove
juice of ½ lemon
2 tbsp olive oil
250 g (7 oz) tomatoes
1 tsp cane sugar
1 tsp black cumin oil
1 tsp pesto

Cut the chilli pod open lengthwise, remove the seeds, then wash and chop finely. Peel and finely chop the spring onion and the garlic. Combine half of each with the lemon juice and 1 tbsp oil, and drizzle over the prawns. Slit the tomatoes, and dip in boiling water for a few seconds. Remove the skins and the seeds, and chop coarsely. Combine with the remainder of the chilli mixture, sugar, and black cumin oil, and season with salt and pepper.

Squeeze the juice from the eggplant, wipe each slice with paper towels, and brush with pesto. Place the eggplant and the prawns on a hot griddle, and brown on both sides. Serve with the tomato and bread.

Good options

You could also cook this dish on a table-top grill, or in a wok. Salmon trout (page 57) and marinated beef (page 51) are also excellent alternatives.

PER PORTION:

180 kcal

10 g protein

12 g fat

8 g carbohydrate

power

Marinated

with spicy fermented wheat liquid

Mussels

Wash the mussels thoroughly, brush them, and carefully remove the beards. Discard any that are open.

Peel the onion and slice into rings. Trim and wash the celery, and cut into sticks.

Heat the oil in a large pan. Glaze the onions, add the celery, and fry briefly. Peel the garlic and crush into the pan. Add the mussels, pour over the fermented wheat liquid, and bring to a boil. Cover with a lid and cook for about 8 minutes. Remove the mussels when all the shells have opened, and keep warm.

Serves two:

1 kg (2 lb 4 oz) mussels
1 onion
1–2 celery stalks
1 tbsp nut oil
1 garlic clove
500 ml (20 fl oz) fermented wheat liquid
75 ml (3 fl oz) sour cream (20% fat)
sea salt and black pepper
1/2 bunch Italian parsley

Pass the cooking liquid through a fine strainer, and reduce to about a third over a high heat. Stir in the sour cream and simmer for another 5 minutes. Season with salt and pepper.

Wash and shake dry the parsley, remove the florets from the stalks, and chop. Sprinkle the parsley over the sauce. Serve with the mussels, accompanied by some bread.

PER PORTION: 225 kcal • 15 g protein • 15 g fat • 8 g carbohydrate

Index

Beauty Food

Abbreviations

tsp = teaspoon
tbsp = tablespoon

Most of the ingredients required for the recipes in this book are available from supermarkets, delicatessens and health food stores. For more information, contact the following importers of organic produce:-
The Organic Food Company, Unit 2, Blacknest Industrial Estate, Blacknest Road, Alton GU34 4PX; (T) 01420 520530 (F) 01420 23985

Windmill Organics, 66 Meadow Close, London SW20 9JD
(T) 0208 395 9749 (F) 0208 286 4732

Fermented wheat juice is produced in Germany by Kanne Brottrunk GMBH
(T) 00 49 2592 97400 (F) 00 49 2592 61370

Note: Fermented wheat juice contains lactic acid. It is a highly alkaline liquid with beneficial, biologically active substances. If the bottled product is not available, pickled cabbage juice can serve as a substitute.

Further information on German food importers is available from The Central Marketing Organisation (T) 0208 944 0484 (F) 0208 944 0441

First published in the UK by
Gaia Books Ltd, 20 High Street,
Stroud, GL5 1AZ

Registered at 66 Charlotte St,
London W1P 1LR
Originally published under the title
Beauty Food

Reproduction: MRM Graphics Ltd,
Winslow, UK.
Printed in Singapore by Imago

ISBN 1 85675 141 4

A catalogue record for this book is available in
the British Library

10 9 8 7 6 5 4 3 2 1

Caution
The techniques and recipes in this book
are to be used at the reader's sole
discretion and risk.
Always consult a doctor if you are in doubt
about a medical condition.

Dagmar Freifrau von Cramm
Dagmar studied ecotrophology, and after
graduation began to practise nutritional
theory in cooking. The mother of three sons,
she has been a freelance food journalist
since 1984. She has been a member of the
Presiding Committee of the German Society
of Nutrition since 1996.
Nutrition advisor: Angela Dowden
Photos: Food Photography Eising, Munich

Susie M. and **Pete Eising** have studios in
Munich and Kennebunkport, Maine/USA.
They studied at the Munich Academy of
Photography, where they established their
own studio for food photography in 1991.